Some Ex

Understanding Personal Independence Payment Benefit

By David P M Wilson

First Edition 2018

Copyright © 2018 David P M Wilson

All rights reserved. No part of this publication may be reproduced, distributed, or transmitted in any form or by any means, including photocopying, recording, or other electronic or mechanical methods, without the prior written permission of the author, except in the case of brief quotations embodied in critical reviews and certain other non-commercial uses permitted by copyright law.

Also available as an e-book for Kindle

Forward

There have been recent changes to the way benefits are awarded over the last few years. We supported a family member through the processes when it was their turn to attend their PIP Assessment. Following on from this, they were turned down and not awarded their PIP benefit, which in our opinion was an incorrect decision.

From this situation we felt prompted to research and learn more about the process, so as to better understand how the system works, and what, if anything, we could do to change their decision. Fortunately, we were successful in our appeal, and this book is based on our experience and research and I write this guide in the hopes that others can gain wisdom and have a smoother journey.

About this Guide

This guide is designed to be a help during what may be a difficult time for you or a member of your family. The guide has been written to be as short and to the point as possible, explaining everything clearly, but not missing out any important details.

Please read through the guide and try and take away the advice within, however remember that legislation can change, and advice from this guide should be taken alongside reading the official guidance given direct from any paperwork produced from the Department of Work and Pensions.

Introduction

<u>Disability</u>
"You're disabled under the Equality Act 2010 if you have a physical or mental impairment that has a 'substantial' and 'long-term' negative effect on your ability to do normal daily activities." (gov.uk). You can review the full text of the Equality Act 2010, however the quote above gives a short simple summary of what disability is and what the expected impact is on someone's life.

A key word from the Equality Act is 'substantial' and this is defined as something which is not trivial. There might be one or more daily tasks which are problematic to complete, such as washing or moving around. However, this isn't the be all and end of being classified as disabled. The nature and impact on one's life can be varied and much harder to pin down in a black and white understanding.

The condition must also be considered long term. Long term is classified as an impairment which has lasted at least 12 months. You automatically meet the disability definition with a HIV or a Cancer diagnosis. In England if you are diagnosed with a terminal illness, the final 6 months of your life, you can be awarded PIP. This is not the case for Scotland and Northern Island where PIP can be awarded following the initial assessment after a formal diagnosis of the life-span limiting condition.

<u>What if I've only just become affected/diagnosed as having an illness, injury, mental health concern or disability?</u>
Each case is different, and the impact on someone's life will vary from person to person. In each instance you

should speak to a health care professional such as the consultant overseeing your care/treatment, your GP or other healthcare professional, for example a Physio Therapist or Occupational Therapist.

What is PIP
Replacing Disability Living Allowance, (DLA) was the Personal Independence Payments (PIP) for people aged 16-64 years old. This change took effect in 2013 and everyone who was receiving DLA, (and are still receiving this benefit), have/are being reassessed in order to decide if they are eligible to receive 'PIP payments'. This money is intended as extra money to help you in your day to day life if you have an illness, disability or mental health condition. It might help top-up wages if you're able to work, or help if you're receiving another type of benefit. Whether you're employed or not does not affect eligibility to receive this benefit. In some special cases the decision as to whether to award PIP was done entirely through paperwork. However, in most cases, it seems that a face to face assessment is required. This is needed to assess and understand what level of support each person needs and as such what level of financial support they would need from the local authority.

If you were not previously receiving DLA, and you're a new claimant, then you will need to contact the Department for Work and Pensions via phone, or via a form only if phone is not suitable for you for health reasons.

Making a Claim for PIP Benefit
The initial information required to make a claim for PIP will be basic information covering the below, ensure

you have it all ready before making the phone call.

- Your personal details and contact details.
- Residency details (also can be known as residency and presence).
- Relevant information relating to any periods spent in Hospital.
- Relevant information relating to any periods spent in Residential Care.
- Claims under special rules for terminally ill people.
- Payment details, so your bank details for the money to go into.
- Information about your illnesses and/or disabilities.

You, the claimant should make this phone call if you're able to, however a support worker, family member or friend can make the call WITH you, but not on their own without you. They will need to pass an identity check first, by sharing some personal details. The claimant should be there with them for the entire phone call.

The DWP will then check basic eligibility conditions, if these are deemed not significant enough for PIP support then a disallowance letter will be issued. If successful, a form called 'How Your Disability Affects You' will be sent out asking for details on how your disability impacts you on a day to day basis. The assessor who reviews your application will need as much detail as possible, and the form you get sent will include what's expected/useful, and what is deemed unhelpful. You should get a response in 2 weeks.

Telling Your Story – Preparing for the assessment.
When you receive your 'How Your Disability Affects You' following the claim phone call. You will need to put down on paper (with help if needed), all information regarding your disability. This should be in your own words and be as clear and accurate as possible. If your condition is fairly stable and has been for years, talk about this, if it new, or has fluctuating elements (eg: some days you struggle to move about your home unaided) then the to be clear about what it's like for you day to day. Talk about bad days, but don't exaggerate or mislead the assessor. You might want to try and explain it as '5 days out of 7 my vision is quite poor, the rest of the time I'm able to see enough to get on with tasks'.

It's important you consider what supporting evidence you can send, by this I mean any paperwork which gives information about how you are personally impacted by your disability. Due to how far and wide disability is, you will be able to tell if a certain document is unsuitable. It shouldn't be anything too general, and will need to give specific information. The DWP discourages you trying to acquire paperwork which you will need to pay for, and likely wait for, as this can delay you getting your claim form back to them. Examples of this may include a letter from your GP. If the DWP wants a letter from your GP, they will request this themselves directly.

Information can be up to 2 years old as long as it is still relevant to your condition today. Only send photocopies, not the originals, and use the same envelop that you will use to send the 'How Your Disability Affects You' form back.

Putting in the effort to provide as much information as possible will aid the decision-making process, and allow the system to work for you much quicker. It may also remove the need for a face to face assessment if one is not necessary.

Information the DWP will want to see. Don't worry if you haven't got any or all of items from the list. Just find what you can, and send in a photocopy.

Reports and Information about you from:
• Specialist professionals
• Community Psychiatric Nurses
• Social workers
• Occupational Therapists
• GPs
• Hospital doctors
• Physiotherapists
• Support workers

Test Results:
• Scans
• Diagnostic Tests
• Audiology

Other papers:
• Your hospital discharge or outpatient clinic letters.
• Your statement of special educational needs.
• Your certificate of visual impairment.
• Your current repeat prescription lists.
• Photographs or X-rays.
• Letters about Other benefits.
• Letters from support workers, family and friends or other people who know you and can provide details of your

disability and the affect it has on you.

<u>Paperwork not to send</u>:
Often with treatment you'll be given leaflets and information to help you and your family better understand your condition such as Type 1 Diabetes or Lupus. These are great general sources of information however they are not acceptable to the DWP assessment process, as they are not specifically about you. Do not include these or similar general documents.

Also do not send letters about future appointments or appointment reminder cards, these again will not be helpful in the application.

A health professional will then review your claim. If they require further information, they will make the arrangements to get this. In most cases a face to face assessment will be needed.

The assessment is carried out by a worker from within the Department of Work and Pensions (DWP), and the Personal Independence Payments (PIP) applicant is assessed off two areas of need:
1) Daily Living
2) Mobility

Daily living: There are ten criteria for daily living:
• Preparing Food
• Eating and Drinking
• Managing your Treatment
• Washing and Bathing
• Managing your Toilet Needs
• Dressing as Undressing

- Communicating
- Reading
- Mixing with People
- Making Budgeting Decisions

Mobility: There are only two criteria for mobility
- Planning and Following a Journey
- Moving Around

Prior to your assessment it would help very much if you and the person accompanying you (if relevant) went through each of these criteria, and thought about what you can do for yourself, what you struggle with, and what you are completely unable to do for yourself.

The assessment will take place in an office building, and you'll need to find the address you will have been sent prior. When you arrive present yourself at the reception, and you'll be shown to a waiting room. The assessor will call you through when it's your turn. You'll likely find that the assessment takes place in a fairly standard looking office, with the assessor sitting behind a desk and typing notes while you answer questions. The assessor will talk you through what you'll be doing over the next half an hour or so, and try to ensure you understand the process. If any part of it is unclear, ask for clarification. The assessor you meet will not be making the final decision, as their job is to simply complete their paperwork by gathering information about you for the report. The report will then go to someone else who will make the decision.

The assessor will assess your claim in two ways. One, by talking to you and asking questions about how you spend your time. They will be interested to hear about your day-to-day life. If you work full or part-time & what you do for a job. The assessor will want to know about how you get on at home. Do you use any aids or special equipment, has there been any modifications made to your home? They'll also be interested in how you get on, out and about in the community, eg: going shopping for groceries. Whether you attend any support groups, hobby clubs and if you do any voluntary work.

The assessor will be looking for your response to certain statements, these are called descriptors. It is then up to the assessor to determine which descriptor matches your ability. For example: "Can read and understand basic and complex written information either unaided or using signs, spectacles or contact lenses." Scores 0 points against Reading. Whereas if the statement: "Needs prompting to be able to read or understand basic written information." Would score you 4 points against this criteria.

It's vitally important to be honest, and it's great to celebrate all you've achieved and can do. However, you must also be clear about your needs. Don't shy away from talking about the areas of your life that need support, no matter how small. The assessor needs a full picture of your life, and they can only gain this by you sharing honestly and in detail. In each case, always use examples of the impact your disability or illness has your day to day life.

The second way they will assess your claim during the meeting is by visually studying you. They will observe how you enter room, the way you speak and articulate yourself while they ask the questions. They'll observe how you are dressed and how you present yourself. It's imperative to show yourself in a normal outfit on a normal day. It's unhelpful to attend smartly dressed then state you struggle to dress yourself, for example. Again, be clear with the assessor, if you have a fluctuating condition, and you find yourself on a good day, share this with them. Eg: If you are stating that you struggle to get in and out of chairs, the assessor will be watching how you climb in and out of the chair in the assessment.

The assessment will cover each one of the criteria previously listed. The criteria have been broken down and expanded upon in the next section. Not all sections will apply to you, however the different points may trigger aspects of your life you never considered.

The assessment is based on points scoring against each criteria of the assessment. The assessor will score you while meeting with you in the assessment. An example of how the points are scored is, if you need help from someone else to wash your hair, you'd score two points. If you need help from someone else to get in and out of the shower, you'd score 3 points. Each criteria is scored to a maximum of 8, 10 or 12. If you score a total of 8 or higher with one of the sections you'll receive the standard rate of PIP, if you score 12 or higher, you'll get the enhanced rate of PIP benefit.

You should certainly prepare some notes about each point and be prepared to speak about what aspects of your life cause you to struggle. You may find it helpful to try and score yourself on each point, I've included the maximum score for each criteria. You may also wish to ask a family member, friend or support worker to go through the points and score you as well.

Assessment Section 1: Daily Living
• Preparing food (scored out of 8)
-Are you able to understand the process of opening food packets/containers?
-Can you open packets/containers such as tin cans, sachets, ready meal boxes and bags?
-Can you peel vegetables etc…
-Are you able to follow instructions to prepare simple meals such as beans on toast, either through memory or by reading/following verbal instructions?
-Do you use any aids or special equipment (other than normal kitchen equipment) to help you prepare food?
-If you are unable to prepare food unaided, think about what barriers there are. Being able to talk about these within the assessment will help them gain a fuller understanding of your abilities.

• Eating and drinking (scored out of 10)
-Are you able to eat unaided? If not, what aids or support do you require?
-Are there some types of food you struggle with more than others. (Runny texture, chewy texture, finger food)
-Do you need your food preparing in a certain way? (Pre-chopped, fork mashed, laid out in a certain way?)
-Can you drink unaided? Any support required?
-Any swallowing issues?

• Managing your treatment (Scored out of 8)
-Can you name any or all of the medication you are on? (If on any medication)
-Do you know what each item of medication is for?
-Are you able to administer the medication yourself as per the pharmacy directions?
-Do you remember to take all your medication? (Right

day, right time, right dose etc...)
-Do you need prompting to take your medication?
-Do you use any aids to help you, remember to take the medication.
-Are there any side effects from one or more of the medications which have an impact on your day to day life (eg: makes you sleepy)

• Washing and bathing (Scored out of 8)
-Are you able to independently wash or bathe at least three times per week?
-Are you able to wash or bath daily?
-Has there been any modifications made to you bathroom to support you to be more independent?
-If you use special equipment, aids or support, to what extent do you require them?

• Managing your toilet needs (Scored out of 8)
-Are there any factors preventing you from completing a visit to the toilet entirely without support, if so, what are they?
-Has there been any modifications to you bathroom, or WC to help you?
-Do you require the presence of another person for all or any part of a visit to the toilet?
-Are you able to use public toilets while on a day out? Do you need to always use disabled toilet facilities?

• Dressing and undressing (Scored out of 8)
-Are you able to dress yourself unaided ensuring you are wearing underwear and one layer of clothing?
-Do you need to wear a certain type of clothing such as jogging bottoms, for the purposes of ease of putting on/removing due to physical disability or sensory needs?

-If you struggle with any aspect of dressing and/or undressing, think about examples of what troubles present themselves.

• Communicating (Scored out of 12)
-Are you able to communicate verbally, being able to greet people, express YES & NO, or speak simple sentences or single words?
-If you are none-verbal, what do you use to communicate? (Sign Language, Makaton, PECs etc...)
-Can you communicate simple information to another person?
-Can you understand simple spoken sentences?
-How are you socialising with peers, are you confident, anxious etc…?
-The assessor will draw a lot of their information regarding this point simply from how to you communicate with them throughout the assessment. However if there are aspects of communicating you want noted, be sure to share this with them.

• Reading (Scored out of 8)
-Can you read simple sentences off the page?
-Can you read in your head or out loud the PIP appointment letter, and explain what it means?
-Do you require alternative reading formats such as large print, braille, audio etc...?
-If reading is difficult for you for whatever reason, what are you able to do for yourself?
-If reading is difficult for you for whatever reason, what do you require from others to help you?
-Is there anything in your life which is made harder due to reading difficulties? (eg: travelling on the bus, understanding utility bills etc…

- Mixing with people (Scored out of 8)
  - How are you around your family (fully confident and involved, anxious, struggles to join in)?
  - Do your family need to make any changes to how they speak, behave etc... to help support you to be more involved?
  - How are you with none family members such as peers?
  - Do you attend social groups or hobby/interest clubs?
  - If you go shopping how are you around members of the general public?
  - Are there any mental health, visual impairment or sensory impairment issues which make any of the above difficult?

- Making budgeting decisions (Scored out of 6)
  - Are you able to plan how money will be allocated across a 30 day period, on things such as bills, groceries and other essential expenses?
  - Are you able to keep on top of your finances?
  - From memory can you state to the nearest £100 what your monthly income is?
  - Do you ever struggle or find yourself without enough funds for essentials such as bills or groceries?
  - Do you ever need to borrow money from family or friends?
  - Do you fully or partly self-fund at least one holiday away from home per year (on your own or with others)?
  - If you need help with budgeting, in what way are you supported?
  - Do you struggle with impulse buying, perhaps as a coping strategy for any mental health concerns?

Assessment Section 2: Mobility:
- Planning and following a journey (Scored out of 12)

-Can you independently prepare a trip to the nearest shopping complex or town/city?
-If you use public transport, do you require any support to get to and from your destination?
-If you need to get to a hospital appointment, are you able to prepare and travel there unaided?
-If there is an event, such as a wedding or birthday party at a new location you haven't ever been to before, how would you find planning the trip?
-Do you feel anxiety at the thought of making trips either to familiar or unfamiliar locations?
-If you require support to plan and or make a journey, what form does this support look like?

•Moving around (Scored out of 12)
-Are you able to walk 200 meters unaided?
-Do you use any aids such as a wheelchair, walking stick, cane (visual impairment), guide dog etc…
-Are you able to move around you home ok?
-Are there any health issues which pose a risk to your safety while moving around?
-Are there any sensory impairment issues which mean certain environments can be tricky to move around?

Additional things to consider
-Is there anything you wish you could do but can't? If so, what is the reason why?
-Have there been times you've had to stop, or felt you've been excluded from something because of your disability?
-Are there any other examples of obstacles in your day to day life which come to mind?

When attending the assessment please consider the points previously raised and present yourself in as true a reflection as you can. The assessment is a safe place to talk about what your needs are, whether it a physical disability, mental health problem or an illness which has affected and is affecting your day-to-day life. You may find it helpful, or at least reassuring to take a family member, friend or Health Support Worker with you. They can either attend simply as a support while you participate in the assessment, or they may wish (with your consent) to speak and contribute into the discussion. They might be helpful to you simply to prompt you on certain aspects of your needs, this can allow the assessor to gain a more accurate picture of you.

After the PIP Assessment
Once the assessment is complete, you will receive the outcome via a letter in the post. The letter will be clearly laid out, giving well-presented details of how the assessor came to their conclusion. You will find each criteria and the score they awarded you for each point. The higher the score, the greater the need for support.

Following this there will be a written report from the assessor talking about the discussion they had with you, what they observed and why the decision was made. If you have deemed the application successful, there is no further action you need to take. Your PIP will be transfers into your allotted account on the date stated in the letter.

My PIP Claim Was Unsuccessful / I will not receive the amount I expected
In the event that your PIP assessment is unsuccessful or you will not be awarded the amount of money you expected. A date in the next month or so will be identified

when the funding will cease if you were previously on DLA, or when the new payment level will commence. However, do not worry too much at this stage. The initial PIP assessment was the first part of three stages from which you can apply for your benefit money. The outcome letter will give some details of the next process should you wish for the decision to be looked at again.

Mandatory Reconsideration

This is the part of the process which PIP candidates can proceed with if the application is declined. There will be some work to do to prepare for this, however a Mandatory Reconsideration is not a particular complicated process to initiate, you will just need to take some time to work on it.

Firstly, it's understandable to feel upset, worried or stressed about this. Anyone facing uncertainty about finances would feel this way. Find someone you trust to speak about how this has made you feel, and perhaps let them read the outcome letter as well, as another person's thoughts will be very helpful moving forward. Give yourself some time to come to terms with what has happened as the next stage will require you to be as level headed as you can.

Read and digest the scores for each section from the outcome letter. Do you feel you were awarded a high enough score for each or any criteria? Reflect on the assessment and think back to what you said or did not say, was there anything further you could had added? If you made notes prior to the assessment compare this to the scoring.

Secondly, read the written report which gives details on what the assessor understood of your needs. They will share about what they made of the questions you answered and their observations of how you appeared throughout the assessment.

The unfortunate fact is that they are only seeing a brief snapshot of you and your life during the assessment. They are basing a decision which has a large impact on your life from spending only a short period of time with you. However, research shows that more than half of PIP decision are changed following a Mandatory Reconsideration, and the PIP money is awarded. (Citizens Advice Bureau)

Preparing a PIP Mandatory Reconsideration
The process you'll need to go through now need not be overly complicated, however I would strongly advise you bring in the support of either a family member, friend or support worker to help you prepare the information you will be submitting.

You will only have ONE Month to submit your Mandatory Reconsideration request from the date of the outcome letter. ACT NOW, do not delay.

Read the outcome letter carefully, and keep it in a safe place, you'll need it.

There is an online form for completing which can be accessed from the government website using a simple internet search.

Mandatory Reconsideration Supporting Letter
I would also suggest completing a letter addressed to the PIP Assessor who will be reviewing your initial assessment. In your letter go back over the different criteria and compare your scoring from before the assessment with how the assessor scored you. Are there any areas you reached which had similar scores, or points which you felt under scored on? Write about examples which make you feel as though you were scored

inaccurately. Read the body of text which will hopefully shed some light onto how the assessor felt about your need for support.

Once this is complete you will hopefully have an idea of the aspects of your support needs which didn't show through at the assessment. You'll really need to think about some further detail and certainly come up with examples of why you deserve a higher score in particular areas.

If you perhaps felt under scored in 'Mixing with People' consider times when you felt overwhelmed by the situation around you. Did you struggle to communicate, or were your particular needs not catered for?

Do you struggle with any day to day tasks?
  -Washing
  -Feeding
  -Moving about
  -Managing your medication or treatment?

Do you struggle with seeing/hearing
  -Understanding what is said to you?
  -Understanding what is happening around you?

Do you use any special equipment or aids in your day to day life? If so how much/often?

It's hard to take a truly unbiased view of yourself. Everyone will find that hard. But now that you're in receipt of a document which shares how you came over in the assessment, it makes the process much easier to build further evidence of what your needs are.

Example PIP Mandatory Reconsideration Letter written by a family member.

(Your Name)
(Your Address & phone number)
Request for a Mandatory Reconsideration
(Your reference number, listed at top of outcome letter)
(Todays date)

Dear Sir/Madam,

I am writing on behalf of (Your Name).

(Name) suffers from mental health issues which include bipolar and depression and as such have affected her for over 20 years. The impact on her life means that she struggles to engage with unfamiliar people confidently in conversation and struggles to articulate/represent herself well in certain situations. (Name) brought her son, (Son's first name), along to the meeting, as a support and to aid the relief of the anxiety she felt in the build-up. Without him she would have been nowhere near as able to speak and function well enough to properly represent herself.

Due to her mental health illness over the years, (Name) does struggle with emotional control, and can demonstrate a reduced tolerance to stress, as well as become upset when faced with unplanned situations which she deems intimidating. It is a shame that after building up to the meeting, and preparing herself to participate in the process, that her mental health needs were not evident to yourself.

To respond to aspects of the assessment letter. (Name) lives very close to the town centre, and part of the assessment I understand, was regarding her ability to plan and travel a route into town. (Name) lives less than five minutes' walk from the town, and is very familiar with the route and due to being unable to work, partly fills her time with walks into town as well as walks to close by family homes. Should (name) be placed in a position to travel to another town, or somewhere unfamiliar, (name) will require the assistance of a family member to drive her.

(Name) also struggles with basic budgeting decisions, and part of her mental health issues are helped by keeping busy and getting out of the house for walks, including walks to the shops. Unfortunately, (name) has never demonstrated a good ability to plan and save money. This prevents her from considering her future needs and building up savings. When (name) is required to save up for something, her family need to ask her for the money on a semi-regular basis which they hold onto until the fund is sufficient, then support her to make the purchase. Examples of this would include (example) & (example). (Name) also struggles to keep on top of her personal paperwork and requires her parents to hold onto her passport and other essential documentation.

It is most unfortunate that (name) was unsuccessful in her interview for the PIP review. However please do process and mandatory reconsideration for (name) as despite coming a long way over the last 20 years, she is unable to mentally and emotionally cope with a lot that life can throw at her.
Yours faithfully

(supports first and second name)
(relationship to PIP applicant)

Writing with and on behalf of (Your full name)

- - - Example Letter End - - -

I have known some people to submit doctors' letters listing diagnoses along with their Mandatory Reconsideration form and cover letter. The notes put together by the DWP state that items like these will not affect the review, however, if you're able to get GP letter without delaying your request, (remember you only have one month to submit your request for a Mandatory Reconsideration!) then there's no harm in sending that as well and may actually be read by the assessor anyway.

Once you have everything ready, perhaps ask someone who knows you to review what you've put together, does it ring true? Do not in any way submit information that is misleading or untrue.

Once you are happy with what you've prepared, send it to the address your outcome letter gives, and await a reply. The wait time could be 1 to 2 months, so you'll need to be patient. You should also make arraignments for how you will cope without the DLA/PIP money if this was due to stop or be reduced.

Outcome: Successful
Once the Mandatory Reconsideration Outcome Letter comes through, this will give you details on how your application was received and what the assessor did with this new information. As stated before, the odds of a positive outcome are in your favour. Keep copies of all letters and a copy of what you sent yourself. This information could be helpful in the future. You do not

need to do anything further, as details of any payment increases and back payments will be mentioned on the letter.

Outcome: Unsuccessful

If the outcome letter states that your claim has been unsuccessful following the Mandatory Reconsideration, it's time to look into the 'Appeal Process'. Please remember you must have gone through a Mandatory Reconsideration first before pursuing an Appeal with the DWP.

Appealing the Decision

The appeal process is when three independent professionals who don't work for DWP look at your claim paperwork to see if they believe the right decision was made. Appeals can take longer than the initial assessment and the mandatory reconsideration process. This may lead to a period of waiting, and with that raised stress levels.

When it comes to the appeals process there is, unfortunately, more work to be done. Please be aware you have 1 month to submit an appeal, so don't delay.

You will receive two copies of the outcome from the Mandatory Reconsideration letter, you'll need one of these copies plus the SSCS1 Form, which you can access from the Government website.

Following the submission of these forms requesting an appeal, you'll receive an HMCTS from DWP which gives details of why they reached the decision they did.

You'll be issued with a date for the hearing, and it's important you prepare for this. Gather absolutely everything you can with regards to letters, paperwork, reports etc... which may help your case and submit these in preparation for the hearing. Get these into order, and work with someone who can help you get ready for the date. It's vitally important you or the person supporting you can find the papers if asked as it can only help the process to have copies with you on the day.

Your appeal (also called a Hearing) will take place in front of a panel called a Social Security Tribunal. As said before this will be three independent experts, who do not know you, and will not have been involved in any of process prior to the appeal being submitted.

SSCS1 Form
This form is divided into sections each requiring particular information from you. The important section to give extra time and attention to is Section 5. This section asks for you to give the reason (or reasons) why you think the decision was wrong. Give as much detail as possible here, just as with the Mandatory Reconsideration, list clear examples.

You or someone supporting you, may have prepared a letter in support of your PIP Mandatory Reconsideration. If so, I suggest reusing this letter and replacing any reference to 'Mandatory Reconsideration' with 'Appeal'. Try to build upon what was written, and see if there is anything new you could add, or any rewording that could be edited in to make it read any better. Asking a new person with a fresh set of eyes to proof read the material would certainly be a helpful move.

Print this out and send with the Form plus any other photocopies of supporting evidence. If you have missed the deadline for requesting an appeal, you must mention this in the covering letter, and state the reason why, (eg: unwell, difficulties with opening post etc…)

Section 6 asks you to choose between attending the hearing in person, or for the hearing to happen without you and based purely on the paperwork you submit. It can certainly be daunting to think about attending some called a 'hearing', and many may choose the paper only hearing on this basis. However, choosing to attend in person, will allow a dialogue between yourself, your supporter and the three experts. They will be able to hear about how your disability affects you in your own words, and also ask any questions they may have. If you find yourself at the point of needing to request an appeal, I would absolutely recommend attending on that basis. The appeal will be entirely centred around you, and all efforts will be made to make it as comfortable for you as possible. The experts will want to meet the real you, not a nervous, overwhelmed individual who is struggling to share their story for fear of where they are. It's a waste of your time and theirs.

These concerns may be eased a degree by section 7 which requires you to specify any dates you will not be able to attend the hearing. Keep this to only dates you really can't reschedule, if you make it too difficult to find a date, this won't help the process. Questions 2, 3 and 4 of section 7 ask about any special requirements you may need such as wheelchair access, hearing aid loop etc… Please use this to help them help you if there are special adjustments you need to make. This may help reduce any stress by removing certain aspects of the hearing which could weigh on your mind.

<u>Preparing for the Hearing.</u>
Once the request and supporting paperwork has been sent in, you wont normally hear anything for 3-4 weeks, but you should be given at least 14 days' notice.

You may wish to consider seeking professional help with the appeal. If so read through the papers sent through from the DWP. This can be a long document, and you'll need to work through to find the parts specifically relevant to you and why they reached the decision they made. See if what they've said rings true, if it does, why not. Record this down for inclusion in the hearing.

Preparing you own statement will help the tribunal to fully hear 'Your Story'. Get someone who knows you well to help prepare this, and in a way that either you can share yourself, or that the person supporting you can read on your behalf.

Another good move is for you to look at obtaining any further useful evidence, this may be a letter from your doctor, social worker, support worker etc… This again is useful for the tribunal process. The most helpful papers you can prepare and take are ones which speak directly about how your disability affects you, particularly relating to the PIP criteria listed previously & included in your PIP outcome letter. Your GP may wish to chare you for this, so its up to you to speak with them and let them know what it is for and to what extent the information needs to go into.

Once you've gathered everything you think you'll need, ask the supporting person to read through it and together consider if each piece of paper helps or hinders your case. Perhaps a letter from a professional has been worded poorly and actually paints you in a more able light than you really feel is true. If so then this material isn't worth including in the submission, however at the tribunal, if they ask if there is any evidence you have but have chosen not to submit, you must tell them about it. Always be truthful to the best of your knowledge and all stages throughout the process.

Finally, when you have the date, and know who, if anyone, will be going with you. Check to ensure you know where you will be going, how you'll get there, and if you can afford to get there. Don't add additional stress on the day by struggling with the journey. You may even wish to practice the trip and find the exact building a day or two before.

Attending the Hearing
Ok, so the day has finally arrived. Hopefully you've chosen to attend and are prepared with notes, copies of paper evidence and a personal statement about how your disability affects you. It's important to remember that the hearing will be tailored to getting the best out of you. It won't be like going for a job interview or being in court. If at any point you feel like you need to pause the meeting, you have the right to ask for a short break. You may wish to leave the room and take a quick stroll, or speak to the person supporting you about anything of concern.

It's also worth noting that there is no point in dressing up formally, or putting any extra special effort into your appearance. As said before you need to present the 'normal' you, and the panel will get a better idea of who you are if you're dressed in normal clothing, and behaving more in keeping with your character.

As with most appointments, you'll need to arrive in plenty of time, and will be shown to a waiting room prior to you time slot. When called through the hearing will take place in what will look more like an office, with those attending probably dressed in normal smart casual clothing. The three experts will greet you and explain the process to you before you all begin. Remember, they do not work for the DWP. One person will be chairing the hearing, while the other two are contributing to the hearing process. One will be a Doctor and the other an expert on disability.

As with everyone on the planet, no one can guarantee that each person is having a good day. The process should be friendly, and the people welcoming, however if you feel this isn't the case, it's perfectly ok to speak up and say that you are being made to feel uncomfortable. If they are not told, they may not realise.

The same can be said for you. Your illness may be affecting you worse than normal that day, or it may be a generally good day for you, health wise. Remember just as with the original PIP Assessment, the panel will be watching you from the moment you enter the room. If you've stated you have mobility issues they'll be watching for signs of this, especially as you enter and exit the room. If you're having a good day, and feel able to move about easier than normal, remember to state this to them.

To give balance to the process, the DWP may send someone to the hearing to explain why they made the decision they did. However, this person is only there to help make the DWP's side of the decision clear, they will not be the person who made the decision and will not push for the DWP's original decision to be upheld.

Remember to take your time 'Telling Your Story', the panel will listen to you, and likely only speak to ask questions for clarity. Read your statement, and hand over all evidence you have brought with you. Be truthful throughout the entire process. If you have chosen to have someone accompany you to share and give evidence, the panel may ask this person to step outside while they speak to you on your own. Don't worry, just remain calm, and answer each question honestly. They will invite the person back in to contribute their input afterwards. If the person has come purely for emotional support, they will not be asked to leave, but may not permitted to address the panel directly during the hearing apart from speaking words of encouragement direct to you.

The questions the panel ask will be to gain as full an understanding of you as possible, if they ask a question and you don't hear it completely, or don't understand what they've asked, ask them to repeat or rephrase. Never give an answer to a question you don't understand, and never simply agree so as to get the question over and done with. It may be that while working through your case they make statements about their understanding of your needs. If at any point you don't agree with what they'd said, speak up and tell them that it is untrue or not quite right. Eg: "You don't have any problems with budgeting and choosing how to spend your money." If it's not true, speak up and put the record straight.

Always try to be clear and confident in sharing exactly what your struggles are, if you required extra help to get to the hearing today, say so. If you need help with your weekly grocery shopping, talk about it. There's no point in being proud or hiding away from the needs you have.

You'll likely never see these people again in your life, so don't be embarrassed or shy. If there are aspects of your life and difficulties you have which don't get covered by the questions, bring these up, and share about them in detail. Everything you add, even if the conversation goes off at a tangent will help your case. I would suggest again making notes, and ticking these off one by one as they are covered. If you were to leave the hearing, and suddenly realise that a whole aspect of your needs weren't discussed, you may have missed an opportunity which could have had an impact on the outcome.

If you have an illness or needs which fluctuate over time, speak about this and be clear that you go through seasons, or that your disability affects you differently one day to the next, have examples ready of what the very bad days look like, and also the better days. Try to give time scales to this, eg: 'My health is worse 4 day out of the normal week. On these days I really struggle to get out the house.'

Adding to this, don't make things up, or exaggerate your needs. Honesty throughout is vital to the benefit system helping those who need it. If they think you are embellishing the truth, this won't help things move in your favour.

The panel will likely make their decision that same day. You will be asked to go to the waiting room while the panel talk among themselves and work through any further discussions regarding your case. You will hopefully not be kept waiting too long and they will share their decision with you, and also give you this decision in writing. If they are unable to reach a decision that day, they will send you their decision in writing in the post in the following week or so.

So that's it

We've covered the three stages of the PIP Assessment. If you or someone you know if going through this, or is about to undergo a PIP assessment, perhaps this guide can be of help. Remember things can change from time to time so always check directly with information from the Department for Work and Pensions.

If you were unsuccessful in each stage, and not awarded any PIP. Do what you can to fully understand why this was ruled to be a suitable outcome. Is it that you simply do not need it with your level of dependence? Or has it been a misruling by those assessing you? You are at any stage, (even after an unsuccessful Hearing) able to seek professional advice. There are likely other benefit packages which could be looked into. Visit your local Citizen's Advice Bureau and see what suggestions they can make.

This guide was written from my experience supporting a family member, and includes research conducted during the process as well as further research following its conclusion when I decided to write this book to help others. I do hope that it was helpful, and that whatever circumstances caused to you pick up this book reach a positive conclusion.

Terms of Reference:

Department of Work and Pensions (DWP)
The government department who oversee and manage all legal and administrative aspects of the British citizens in the workplace, pensions and the benefits system.

Personal Independence Payments (PIP)
The name of the benefit paid to all those 18 and over who require extra financial support because they are unable to work, or find it harder to work.

Adviser
This is an expert who gives advice about the process and your claim. This person might also be able to help you prepare for, and understand the hearing process. They may even be able to represent you.

Mandatory Reconsideration
This is the part of the process which follows the initial assessment. If you request a Mandatory Reconsideration, it means you don't agree with the outcome of the assessment, and wish to add some further information and get it looked at again. Remember, this process isn't automatic, and you have 1 month to request this. You must request a Mandatory Reconsideration before you can request an Appeal.

Appeal
This is the process which following a Mandatory Reconsideration, and means you don't agree with the outcome. A date will be booked for a panel of three experts who do not work for DWP to look at the

claim and decide if the right result happened. If they think the wrong decision was made, they will change it.

Carer
This is a person who helps and supported people who need additional help due to illness or disability. They will likely be involved in day to day care or at least involved several times per week. It may be somebody provided by the local authority, or from a charity. You might also employ someone to support you. This person could also be your partner, a member of your family, or a friend. The help they offer will depend entirely on your needs and might be as simple of doing some tidying up around your home, prompting you to do things, or be something more such as giving you physical support to complete day to day tasks such as washing or going shopping.

Hearing
When your appeal is looked at by a Tribunal of experts. This is something you must prepare for, and I strongly advise you attend in person and give a face-to-face account of your needs. A hearing like this isn't as scary as it may seem, don't be put off by the name. 69% of people who request a tribunal are successful and get the original decision overturned (Mirror.co.uk, March 2018)

SSCS1 Form
This is the name of the form you must complete in full to ask for an appeal. You can access this from the government website with a simple internet search.

Frequently Asked Questions

<u>What if my Disability or Illness has got worse since I made my original application?</u>
If your illness or disability has got worse since the date of your application and you were refused benefit altogether, you are entitled to make a new claim. If you were given some benefit but not as much as you think you should get, you need to ask for your benefit to be reassessed.

<u>My disability or illness has become better since I was successful in getting PIP benefits.</u>
You must inform the DWP and update them on your condition. The PIP will be reviewed, and the amount adjusted. You may need to go in for a new assessment. Do not simply continue to take PIP benefits if you are no longer in need of it.

<u>I've missed the deadline for requesting a Mandatory Reconsideration or Appeal.</u>
If the deadline is about the pass, you are able to request a Mandatory Reconsideration over the phone, however its always best done in writing if time allows. If the deadline has completely passed by up to two weeks, still submit your request and state a reason (excuse) as to why it is late. Eg: You may need help opening and dealing with post, or the emotional stress involved had a negative impact on your mental health.

If longer has passed, you will need to think of a suitable excuse as while such a length of time has passes. The DWP can accept this request even if it is late, however they do not have to. 13 months will have needed to have passed before they certainly won't look at the decision again.

<u>I've made an appointment for the Assessment / Appeal, but I can no longer make the planned date.</u>
You will need to phone the DWP or Hearing Office as soon as possible, and ask to rearranged the date. Details will be on your letter.

Reference:

Equality Act, gov.uk website, accessed July 2018

Mirror.co.uk, accessed March 2018

Citizens Advice Bureau

Disclaimer

This book and its contents are the understood process of completing the PIP Assessment, the Mandatory Reconsideration and the Appeals process. Any inaccurate, out of date or wrong information has occurred through genuine error despite the very best efforts of the author and proof readers, and is in no way meant to mislead or confuse the reader. This book should not be used as a stand-alone document, and should be used in conjunction with information from the Department of Work and Pensions UK. The author and publisher cannot be held responsible for any problems which occur from following this book if any aspect of the process has changed, if the reader acted through a misunderstanding of what they read, or if the author misunderstood, or was misled about any part of the process during the research stage. Always follow the advice of DWP staff and any experts working in or for the field of Benefit claims. The author accepts no responsibility for any problems, delays, issues or unsuccessful applications within any of the process which arise from someone using the information in this book correctly or incorrectly. All information believed to be correct at time of publishing.

Printed in Great Britain
by Amazon